The

The purpose of the books in this series is to awaken and kindle your interest in the many natural healing resources available all around you, and to demonstrate how simple, harmless remedies found in nature are often more effective than artificially created chemicals found in your local pharmacy, which may, in "curing" you, bring unpleasant and harmful side effects. By studying the advice given here, you will become acquainted with many hitherto secret, yet easily accessible, remedies from the Swiss folklore of healing which are only waiting to be discovered and put to good use.

The Swiss Nature Doctor's
LIBRARY OF NATURAL HEALTH

HOME TREATMENT OF COMMON AILMENTS
SECRETS OF THERAPEUTIC HERBS
GUIDE TO A HEALTHIER HEART AND CIRCULATORY SYSTEM
RECOMMENDED FOODS FOR HEALTH AND VITALITY
HEALTHFUL ADVICE ON NATURAL DIET
BOOK OF 12 HEALTH-RESTORING TREATMENTS
HINTS FOR A HEALTHIER LIVER
LIVING THE ACTIVE LIFE AT AGE 90
BOOK OF 14 AMAZING HERBAL MEDICINES

For information on this exciting series,
write to the Publisher

The Swiss Nature Doctor's Book Of Twelve Health-Restoring Remedies

Dr. A. Vogel

Keats Publishing, Inc. New Canaan, Connecticut

The Swiss Nature Doctor's Book of 12 Health-Restoring Treatments is not intended as medical advice. Its purpose is solely informational and educational. Please consult a medical or health professional should the need for one be indicated.

THE SWISS NATURE DOCTOR'S BOOK OF 12
HEALTH-RESTORING TREATMENTS

Copyright © 1990 by A. Vogel
All Rights Reserved

No part of this book may be copied or reproduced in any form without the written consent of the publisher.

ISBN: 0-87983-522-2

Published by Keats Publishing, Inc.
27 Pine Street (Box 876)
New Canaan, Connecticut 06840

Contents

Introduction 7
7 General Treatments
Breathing Means Life 7
   The Influence of Correct Breathing on Illness 8
Building Resistance to Disease 8
   Guard Against the Consequences of Infectious Disease 8
   Natural Antibiotics and Immunity 9
Water and Its Therapeutic Effect 9
   Currents of Health 10
   Therapeutic Value of Sea Bathing 10
   Alternating Hot and Cold Water Therapies 10
A Personal Spring Cleaning 11
   The Wild Kitchen 11
"Let Your Food Be Your Medicine" 11
   The Low-Protein Diet 12
Fasting 14
The Remedial Powers of Juices 15
   A Special Curative Juice Diet 15

5 Treatments for Specific Conditions
Asthma and Pulmonary Disease 16
   Bronchial Asthma 16
   Cardiac Asthma 17
   Important Factors in the Treatment of Pulmonary
     Diseases 17
A Diet for Diabetics 18
Arthritis and Rheumatism 18
Seven Basic Rules for the Prevention of Cancer 20
Dealing with Intestinal Parasites 21
Dr. Alfred Vogel—"The Nature Doctor" in Person 23
   Bioforce: Founding and Growth 24

Introduction

In the course of the six decades of my work with natural healing, I have found many approaches to treatment which have been effective, both for specific health problems and for the preservation or restoration of good health in a general way. In this booklet I share with you a dozen of these treatment methods, for your better understanding of the role nature plays in the cure of disease and in the promotion of the well-being that is our birthright. Whether these treatments call for the use of natural foods and plants or for our own efforts to lead a more healthful life, they are founded upon the natural principles which have always been, and continue to be, the basis of my work.

7 GENERAL TREATMENTS

Breathing Means Life

Many years ago, frustration, worry and anger combined with other stresses to impair my health, as manifested by breathing difficulties, heart problems and, to top everything off, appendicitis. A colleague who examined me was concerned and fearful, and advised an operation. Instead, I took some natural remedial measures which brought some slight relief, but the condition did not really improve—what should I do?

I hit upon the idea of exercising the abdominal organs by rhythmic breathing, which soon brought about an improvement, manifested by a peculiar surge of bodily warmth and the disappearance of pains in the heart region. Sleep became more restful and worries, sorrows and anxieties no longer woke me in the middle of the night. From a physical point of view, my abdominal muscles seemed the first to benefit. They became stronger, and my digestion improved.

A notable feature of the breathing exercises I developed was the practice of expanding the abdomen rather than the chest in order to breathe in and contracting the abdomen while exhaling. If this is done vigorously the chest fills up well and in time can hold twice as much air as before.

At the beginning I practiced this breathing exercise briefly once or twice a day, but eventually brought it up to four times a day, 15 minutes at a time.

The Influence of Correct Breathing on Illness. Correct breathing is not only good for the head, abdomen and the whole body, but it influences and stimulates the activity of the sympathetic and parasympathetic nervous systems. Even conditions such as angina pectoris may be improved, as may asthma.

While constipation requires regular intake of natural food for improvement, correct breathing can help. If you follow the breathing exercises I have described for up to fifteen minutes in the morning, afternoon and evening, the bowels will eventually begin to function more efficiently.

For those concerned with slimness, the "spare tire" will disappear more quickly if correct breathing is combined with dietary reform.

Regularity of the exercises is of the utmost importance because it helps the body get used to a new rhythm; we will find that it is better than any other form of exercise. This is a "medicine" that is within reach of everybody and costs nothing but a little effort, concentration and perseverance.

Building Resistance to Disease

Guard Against the Consequences of Infectious Disease. Toxins in the system which stem from infectious disease must be eliminated or they will lead to ill health. Neglected or not fully cured mumps can cause pancreatitis. Improperly treated tonsillitis may give rise to such heart trouble as myocarditis or endocarditis. Many other diseases can arise when toxins remain in the body and are not cleared out. It is therefore important that every effort be made to ensure complete excretion of toxins in cases of infectious diseases. The following three main points must be observed:

1. Elimination through the skin by sweating. Apply hot packs and take hot showers. The saunas and steam baths available at many health clubs are useful for this purpose.

2. Elimination through the kidneys by means of a simple kidney remedy such as goldenrod or parsley tea, or some other available natural means of stimulating the kidneys. Onion poultices are effective, too.

3. Elimination through the bowels. Fever usually tends to dry them up. To stimulate movement, use simple natural remedies like linseed tea, psyllium seed, manna stick tea, soaked figs or prunes. A fruit juice diet without eating anything else is also excellent.

If you pay close attention to these three points, you can avoid the complications often experienced as a result of ineffectively treated infectious diseases.

Natural Antibiotics and Immunity. Rather than dealing with the consequences of infectious diseases, as described above, it would of course be preferable to avoid such diseases entirely! We have seen how many formerly devastating diseases such as influenza have lost their dreadful impact on our society. Some of this is due to medical advances, but it is clear that the processes of nature have come to endow us with an immunity to many conditions that were formerly prevalent, and modern research is showing us that a capably functioning immune system can stave off both infectious and degenerative diseases.

Chemical antibiotics work by destroying pathogenic organisms, and too often in doing so they destroy the health-promoting intestinal flora we depend on. Natural antibiotics both counter disease-producing organisms and build up resistance to disease. Liver patients especially may benefit from these, as may those with weak lungs, cancer and many other serious diseases.

Many years ago I made some interesting experiments with horseradish, watercress, garden cress—and even nasturtiums. I discovered that those who ate these plants regularly became more resistant to disease, particularly colds and infections. I can remember how some people laughed at the idea of nasturtiums having any nutritional or remedial value, but having observed that patients eating them did in fact improve, I continued to use them in my work. Recent work in Germany has established the scientific validity of the nutritional value of nasturtiums. (An extract of nasturtium is also a powerful insecticide, which is suggestive of its overall powers.) Watercress is similar in effect, as I have demonstrated in many experiments. Eat watercress (preferably wild) regularly, and you will feel your resistance to colds, catarrh and other infectious diseases increase.

Water and Its Therapeutic Effect

Traveling in the Americas and the South Sea islands many years ago, I noticed that the natives often bathed in water so muddy that it was black, yellow or red. Much later I took a bath in a mud pond in northern Scandinavia, and when I stepped out of the muddy water I felt really refreshed and began to think about the effect more closely. It suddenly crossed my mind that we apply clay-water compresses because they are better than just water packs. Then it dawned on me that dirty—that is, muddy—water was not so bad after all; I realized that it can still have a therapeutic effect in spite of its uninviting appearance, provided of course that the muddiness is nothing but natural clay or some other kind of earth.

Currents of Health. Some time later an analytical chemist proved to me by means of an apparatus that measures electrical tension that water carries energy that is transmitted to the human body. Not every kind of water has the same electrical field or the same therapeutic effect. Minerals dissolved in the water can add medicinal properties. These substances are usually picked up by the water flowing from the source deep in the earth and passing over mineral deposits. That is what makes it remedial when used as bath water and for drinking.

Therapeutic Value of Sea Bathing. Salt water has an osmotic effect, drawing water from the body. People who always have some water retention in the legs will feel considerably better after bathing in the sea. If you tend to obesity, sea bathing will usually be helpful in weight loss. Overweight and fat can be reduced because the sea stimulates the thyroid and gonads, benefiting the entire metabolism. Sea air and sea bathing are beneficial in cases of circulatory disorders, and diabetics will find sea bathing good for them when they swim a lot and walk along the beach and over the dunes.

Alternating Hot and Cold Water Therapies. Hot and cold water applications are excellent for poor circulation and a fine help in removing congestion.

Apply hot water or herbal packs for about three minutes, then replace with a cold water pack, but leave this on no longer than half a minute. Repeat the hot pack, followed by the cold, then hot again and so on for 20 to 30 minutes. If you take alternating hot and cold baths, you must stay in the cold water only the same number of seconds as you spent minutes in the hot water—10 minutes in the hot water, then 10 seconds in the cold, and so on. This rule also applies to alternating hot and cold foot and arm baths. These applications should never make you feel chilled, but always warm and comfortable.

A Personal Spring Cleaning

However well we manage over the winter, the coming of spring provides us with an opportunity and a challenge to repair and renew our bodily health. What makes it more of a challenge is the phenomenon of "spring fever," a lassitude that makes exertion, even in our own behalf, uncomfortably effortful. There are a number of things you can do to combat spring fever. First of all, increase your physical and breathing exercises. Vigorous walking or hiking will help your body to exhale a substantial amount of accumulated wastes. It may make you sweat, and that is good because it stimulates the skin and helps it to exude toxins. A home sweat bath or sauna, if you have one, will be very helpful—but do not overdo it, especially if you have any kind of heart problem.

The Wild Kitchen. The sudden renewal of nature's bounty in the spring offers us a variety of wild foods to help restore our winter-dampened vitality. Certain spring flowers and leaves make superb herb teas. The bright yellow flowers of coltsfoot can help rid you of winter's phlegm. As soon as the raspberry, blackberry, blackthorn and hawthorn bring forth tender new shoots, gather them to prepare a wonderful, mineral-rich spring tea from their fresh leaves. Do the same with young strawberry leaves and the tender shoots of the birch tree. The country people who have made this spring tea for many generations sweeten it with honey only. Not only do such infusions supply you with nutritive salts, but they stimulate the kidneys, an important aspect of a spring cleansing treatment. Those who take this spring tea regularly are convinced that it purifies the system, purging it of winter wastes and infusing the new energies of spring.

When the stinging nettles have grown large enough, gather some young shoots every day and add them, chopped fine, to your salads; or lightly steamed as a vegetable, they are delicious. Many country people also use another wild salad herb that stimulates the liver, young dandelion leaves. When these are fresh and tender, they should be used in salads every day.

"Let Your Food Be Your Medicine"

This wise saying of the ancient physician Hippocrates provides the firm foundation of much natural therapy. The role of a poor diet in destroying health, and of a good diet in restoring it, cannot be overstated. By adhering to a correct diet we can do much to back up whatever natural remedy or treatment we may take.

There is little point in swallowing medicines or taking water treatments if we pay no attention to the food we are eating. It is useless, for example, to take remedies to prevent the formation of uric acid if at the same time we encourage that formation by eating eggs and other concentrated protein foods. Instead of being guided by our palates, we must consider our food from the standpoint of what it can do for us. It will take persistence to restore health, for did it not require persistence in eating the wrong things to make us susceptible to disease? Yet, given this persistence, many patients have overcome their ailments and recovered their health.

The Low-Protein Diet. This diet is of paramount importance in all metabolic and digestive disturbances, in conditions of high blood pressure, arthritis, rheumatism and gout, and should be followed for a considerable period. Protein is found chiefly in meat, eggs, milk and milk products, peas, beans and lentils; so vegetarians should reduce their intake of milk products and legumes. Meat-eaters should refrain from pork, sausages and cold cuts and restrict the diet to veal, beef, lamb and mutton. Eggs, cheese and dishes prepared with them should also be avoided; but if you must eat eggs, eat few and eat them raw. They can be beaten and added to soup. Eggs produce a good deal of uric acid, and arthritis sufferers are better off without them. Those who like cheese should eat little, and then only the mild types, along with vegetables, for their midday meal. Soft white cheese such as cottage cheese is much better than hard cheese, as it has none of the drawbacks of other high-protein foods and actually assists the functioning of the liver.

And of course, avoid fried foods and all denatured, refined food. Fatty fried foods have no place at all in the diet of anyone with a sensitive liver. To complement a proper diet and support any treatment you are undertaking for your health, you would do well to cut out all white flour and refined sugar products, also all canned food and fruit and any other refined or denatured food items.

Here are some general suggestions for healthy eating throughout the day.

Breakfast. The ideal foundation of a nourishing breakfast is a muesli with apples or fruit in season. Add nuts and whole-grain flakes to enrich it further. A very nutritive addition is whole wheat, soaked and then put through a food mill. Raisins can be mixed with the wheat and chopped in with it; they are excellent for the blood. A level teaspoon of ground linseed may be added if constipation is a problem. Use honey or grape sugar to sweeten.

Whole-wheat or whole-grain crispbread or bread with a little butter, honey or rose hip conserve can follow the muesli; if you like, sprinkle a little wheat germ on the bread or the muesli.

A cup of rose hip tea sweetened with honey or grape sugar is a healthful breakfast drink; if you wish, top it with a little cream or milk. For a change you might like some cereal-based coffee substitute. An occasional fruit juice breakfast is beneficial, and grape, orange or grapefruit juice (which is especially good for the kidneys, liver and entire glandular system) can be recommended.

Midday meal (dinner). Depending on the season, a great variety of salads may be served; the dressing can be prepared with lemon or whey concentrate, but never use vinegar. Another tasty dressing can be made with sour cream or yogurt, and herbs such as savory, marjoram and thyme can add a zesty flavor. Every kind of cabbage is good, but is best eaten raw. Cole slaw is well tolerated, and is tasty, healthful and nutritive.

The next course is vegetables, which, if steamed, should not cause fermentation and consequent flatulence. A third category, starch-containing food, should also be on the menu. From a dietetic point of view, whole rice is best. It has a normalizing effect on blood pressure, and is the best source of carbohydrates. Whole wheat also makes an ideal dish and should be prepared like rice; millet and buckwheat are also good starch foods.

If you like soup, choose vegetable soup, but only mildly seasoned. Meat soups promote the formation of uric acid. For those who like meat, a little beef or veal may be added to the main dish, but it should be kept to a minimum.

A sweet dessert has no place in a health diet because it encourages fermentation. If you cannot overcome your desire for fruit or some other naturally sweet food after the meal, postpone indulging your fancy until at least four in the afternoon.

Slow eating and mixing everything thoroughly with saliva will allow you to gain the maximum value from whatever you eat.

Supper. I prefer this term to dinner for the evening meal, as it should be light, not a heavy main meal. A light meal will be digested before it is time to go to bed. Supper may be the same as breakfast, but it does not have to consist of sweet food and fruit. A good and inexpensive dish is made with ordinary oat flakes, currants or raisins and a modest amount of chopped nuts. Bread or crispbread, as at breakfast, with a little butter or margarine, goes well with a fruit salad.

As a change, a meal of sandwiches and a salad can be enjoyable. You can use your imagination to create a variety of sandwiches. Spread a piece of whole-grain bread or crispbread lightly with butter and just a touch of a vegetable or yeast extract; and to this foundation add cottage cheese mixed with chives, slices of garlic, watercress, tomato, grated carrot with a little horseradish, or whatever your imagination suggests—so long as you let it range only among the foods that are good for you.

In the spring, radishes are a welcome addition to the sandwich menu, but should be used sparingly because they are quite strong and could overstimulate or irritate the liver.

Fasting

One of the best remedies for maintaining general well-being is fasting. If we do not feel well because we ate too much, if our stomach is upset because we have eaten unsuitable food, fasting is the most natural remedy.

An occasional brief fast is a good idea; plan ahead to have a fruit juice day, followed by one or two days of taking only pure water. Before you begin the fast, make sure the bowels are empty; mucilage-producing substances such as psyllium seed or a herbal laxative such as manna will help move the bowels.

If your liver is functioning properly, you can now begin the fruit juice phase with orange, grapefruit or grape juice, according to what is in season. During the berry season, add berries to the list. Any wastes in the body will be eliminated and your organs will begin to function more efficiently. Should you feel sick during the fast, speed up the elimination by encouraging skin function: friction baths, vigorous toweling or brushing down will stimulate circulation, while deep breathing exercises will likewise help to get rid of the feeling of sickness. If you get very hungry, chew a few raisins slowly and thoroughly. The Bedouins wandering in the desert often live on nothing but a few dates a day, because they get the full benefit from this frugal meal by chewing thoroughly and predigesting it properly.

Here is one important rule you must observe: Never enter upon a fast while disturbed, annoyed or worried about something. A happy frame of mind is a natural medicine that stimulates the endocrine glands and keeps them at peak efficiency.

How long should a fast last? That should be determined by individual needs. Two or three days may be sufficient; however, if you have kept it up for three days, it is perhaps a pity to stop. The first three days are like climbing a high mountain; having scaled the hardest part, the worst is over and, to one's surprise, the going becomes easy and enjoyable. So it is after the first three days of fasting. The body has adapted to the change and can easily stand another five days. An eight-day fast, taking only fruit juice, will give your body a complete cleansing. If you suffer from arthritis, you will find it beneficial to continue the fast even longer. As reported in the Scriptures, Christ fasted for forty days. It is an established fact that when great demands are made on the mind, fasting will help to make one's thoughts crystal-clear, one's understanding precise and accurate.

In order to step up elimination of wastes through the urine, it is of paramount importance to drink 1 to 1½ liters (2-3 pints) of weak rose hip, goldenrod or kidney tea daily during the duration of a juice or fast diet.

The Remedial Powers of Juices

In addition to providing an introductory phase to a fast, juices are powerful healing and health-enhancing substances in their own right. Some researchers have suggested that the alkaline properties of raw juices neutralize the free acids in the system and so rehabilitate the mineral metabolism, making successful treatment of gastric ulcers possible. However, the mere knowledge that juices can cure is infinitely more valuable than any scientific explanation advanced in this connection. Today it is easier to convince people because science has confirmed our assertions that raw juices and raw vegetables are wonderful remedies. It is and will remain a fact that the raw juices of potato and cabbage will heal gastric and duodenal ulcers.

Even more interesting is the observation I made in connection with raw potato, cabbage and carrot juices in the treatment of gout, rheumatism and allied conditions. If the juices are taken in conjunction with a strictly natural diet, these diseases often eventually yield to treatment.

Since 1935 I have been prescribing vegetable juices with excellent results. The juices I have used are beet, carrot, cabbage and sauerkraut, either pure or mixed. Whatever the disease concerned, these juices have helped to solve the dietetic difficulties.

A Special Curative Juice Diet. Before breakfast, on an empty stomach, take half a glass of raw potato juice diluted with a little warm water. The breakfast itself should consist of whole wheat that has been soaked in water for a day or two. It can be made more palatable with the addition of vegetable stock or fresh butter. If the bowels need special attention, add psyllium seed or freshly ground linseed to the wheat. Crispbread with butter and wheat germ will complete your breakfast. If the liver is not functioning properly, drink a glass of raw carrot juice. Chew all food well and insalivate it thoroughly.

For the midday meal, add a cup of raw cabbage juice to a hearty vegetable broth after the soup is cooked and off the stove; then a dish of natural brown rice, vegetables and a salad. See the section "Let Your Food Be Your Medicine" for details of the good-health diet in general. As in that diet, supper should resemble breakfast. Keep off fruit on this special diet, using only vegetable juices.

With this diet it has proven possible to relieve a stomach ulcer within a month. Gout and rheumatic complaints should improve within two or three months and slowly disappear. Afterwards, continue with the diet but have only fruit every other day. Avoid all sausages, cold cuts, pork, canned foods, white sugar, white flour and everything made from it—you would in fact do well to forget these items altogether. You may start eating meat again after six months, but only veal or beef.

Since these juices, with the exception of carrot juice, are not very palatable, try mixing them in a thick minestrone soup. The vegetable flavors will neutralize the strong taste of the raw juice. You will have to eat this soup with the raw juices twice a day and have in between meals two additional deciliters (a little less than a cup) of juice. In grave cases, 4 or 5 deciliters daily are absolutely essential.

5 Treatments for Specific Conditions

Asthma and Pulmonary Disease

Bronchial Asthma. This condition is mainly caused by certain climatic conditions, and a change in environment can often bring about a cure. Living by the sea, where the air contains iodine, usually has a positive effect, as, quite often, does high altitude. An elevation of 2800 feet generally suffices, though sometimes one of up to 4500 feet may be necessary to overcome the problem. The third alternative is the hot, dry air of the desert, which has helped to relieve asthmatic disorders.

It is possible that asthmatic spasms are caused by pollen in the air. This "seasonal asthma" in this respect resembles hay fever, which also results from sensitivity to pollen. If your financial situation permits you to move to a different climatic zone, you should by all means do so, since a change of climate together with the appropriate natural remedies should in the course of time lead to a cure of a case of bronchial asthma.

Common practice is to treat asthma with strong remedies, containing ephedrine, atropine or an extract of jimson weed; these are extremely powerful and have a dependency potential. Homeopathic remedies are to be preferred, and herbal remedies containing butterbur have been effective.

Cardiac Asthma. Cardiac asthma is the result of a weak heart. As soon as the problem has been diagnosed, treatment with cardiac remedies and those that influence the vascular system should begin. Instead of medicines containing digitalis, which tend to accumulate in the body, it is recommended to take convallaria (lily of the valley) in connection with sea squill (sea onion). Preparations containing hawthorn and calcium are also helpful.

Important Factors in the Treatment of Pulmonary Diseases. It is strange that orthodox medicine still does not pay enough attention to the basic healing factors in the treatment of lung patients. Much can be achieved by rest, light, air and sun, and their value has been proven beyond doubt, and orthodox medicine honestly admits that it is the climate that provides a cure for lung disease.

But another factor must not be forgotten: nutritional therapy. The body must be supplied with substances in which it is deficient before it can attempt regeneration. First on the list are foods rich in calcium and vitamins; they are indispensable. Raw, freshly pressed carrot juice or raw, finely grated carrots, freshly pressed juice of grapes, oranges, grapefruit and other wholesome juices, should be taken in little sips, slowly and well insalivated. If you observe this advice, the fruit acid will cause no unpleasant gastric disturbances.

The intake of protein foods must be reduced, and natural culinary herbs that stimulate the appetite are recommended. I have always seen excellent results with a calcium-rich preparation derived from nettles, together with herbs containing silica, such as galeopsis. Usnea, the moss or lichen found on larch trees, also deserves special mention; it strengthens the pulmonary system, and can be taken in a tea if chewing the actual lichen presents problems. Cod liver oil or emulsions are recommended, if the patient can take them.

It is of great importance to influence the patient psychologically. Glandular functions must be in order, and this depends a great deal on the state of mind. The skin should be stimulated, too. Give the body a daily brush massage and afterwards apply a good skin oil containing natural herbal ingredients that encourage the function of the skin.

A Diet for Diabetics

Diabetics need to pay special attention to their diet. Unlike other diseases, diabetes makes the patient want to eat more. We must see to it that he gets an adequate amount of food, but with the proviso that it does not contain too many carbohydrates. This can be achieved by giving the diabetic primarily vegetables which are rich in vitamins but low in carbohydrates. If the patient is used to eating meat, he must restrict himself to small quantities of lean cuts. The following menu for one day is presented as an example to follow.

Breakfast. Take your pick of buttermilk, sour milk or cereal-based coffee substitute. For a change, you can sometimes take yogurt. Make sandwiches using rye bread, flake bread, whole-meal bread or crispbread. Spread the bread with soft white cheese such as cottage cheese. Dress the sandwich with tomato slices or kitchen herbs such as parsley, chives or freshly grated horseradish.

If you prefer fruit for breakfast, follow this alternative menu: coffee substitute with cream, fruit muesli with rye flakes, whole rice flakes or an all-bran cereal. Use fresh fruit in season; bilberries (blueberries), black currants and apples are very good. Add sesame seeds or grated almonds, but no sugar. When berries are out of season, use natural fruit juices with no additives.

Midday meal (lunch). Soya mix patties, creamy cottage cheese or curds with horseradish, and a seasonal vegetable, steamed or *au gratin*. A large plate of salad made up of various vegetables is most important; again, the choice is determined by the season. Excellent are cabbage, raw sauerkraut with no additives, lettuce and above all plenty of cress, including nasturtium leaves.

You may have a cup of the cereal coffee substitute with a little cream after your meal; be sure to avoid beverages with chemical additives.

Here is another sample menu for those who like meat: Broiled veal or beef, steamed vegetables, a mixed salad as above.

Evening meal (supper). You would do well to eat only a light meal at night; follow the suggestions given for breakfast. Here is an alternative: Vegetable or sesame soup, a vegetable prepared in the oven or steamed tomatoes, a small plate of mixed salad or raw natural sauerkraut.

Arthritis and Rheumatism

The cause of rheumatoid arthritis is still in dispute, but more often than not we find in association with arthritis some local focus of infection which discharges a constant stream of toxins or pathogenic organisms into the blood; the presence of viruses has also been noted. Nevertheless, no conclusive explanation for the disease has so far been presented.

I have observed that patients suffering from rheumatoid arthritis usually have a family history of gout, arthritis or some other rheumatic disease, suggesting that predisposition is a factor. This would explain why some individuals with the same "triggering" circumstance—say an abscessed tooth—respond by developing arthritis while another may come down with a kidney problem or a circulatory disorder or not be seriously affected at all.

Standard treatment for arthritis is mainly pain relievers and the powerful cortisone derivatives, which are of erratic effectiveness and often have dangerous side effects. I have found that a combination of natural therapies can be extremely effective, and offer this approach for your consideration.

The treatment recommended for cases of arthritis, rheumatism and gout is successful only if followed for at least six months, better still for a full year, cutting out completely any food with excess acidity. Instead, your food must now be highly alkaline, ruling out all meat, fish, eggs and cheese. You can see why this idea does not appeal to everyone, and is often considered too difficult to follow. Yet after a few weeks the patient will not regret having taken the plunge and changed his diet; feeling the aches and pains start to recede makes the sacrifice worth while.

Upon awakening, the first item is invigorating personal hygiene. A warm shower—increase the heat gradually until it is quite hot—followed by a rubdown with some herbal preparation containing comfrey is an excellent start. Breakfast will consist of 3 to 5 tablespoons of high-value muesli; mix in the juice of half a lemon. You can also have half a grapefruit or the juice of two or three mandarin oranges or clementines (seedless tangerines). Next add half a tablespoon of pure honey, three tablespoons of coffee cream or half a tablespoon of almond purée. Instead of apples, mash and add berries when they are in season. In addition to this dish, have one or two slices of whole-grain bread with butter or a good vegetable margarine. A cup of rose hip tea is excellent as a mild stimulant for the kidneys.

Lunch is prepared without any frying, for the benefit of the liver. For every meal it is enough to have a 100 percent natural food containing starch, such as brown rice, potatoes, millet, buckwheat, corn or soya. An accompanying vegetable should be steamed, then browned without fat in an earthenware pot in the oven. Leeks, fennel, zucchini, eggplant, cabbage stems and kohlrabi are among the vegetables suitable for this treatment. Tomatoes—

preferably grown in your own garden and ripened on the plant—should be eaten raw in salads. Fresh green peas and beans supplement the protein foods.

Salad vegetables have healing properties. According to the season, use cress, dandelion shoots or lamb's lettuce; coleslaw, raw sauerkraut and carrots are highly valuable.

For your beverage, choose a good mineral water without gas, or an all-natural mixed vegetable juice. The total food intake at each meal should be moderate; as a matter of fact, when eating whole foods, it is possible to eat 40 to 50 percent less than one is accustomed to, yet be both satisfied and better nourished.

The evening meal should be similar to the breakfast; a lighter meal is easier to digest and promotes restful sleep.

If you want to speed up the treatment, go on a vegetable juice diet for one or two days a week. Take one liter (2 pints) of juice during the day, sipping it regularly every hour.

Now and then during the treatment have your urine tested so you can see what is eliminated from your body. This is one measure of the success of the treatment, as improvement depends upon the acid-alkaline balance being restored.

Seven Basic Rules for the Prevention of Cancer

The following seven rules will give you an idea of the effective precautionary measures you can take to prevent cancer as far as possible. You should be aware of them all the time.

Rule One. We live in restless, uneasy times with many failures and disappointments, but if we let worries and anxieties dominate us, we should not be surprised if our health begins to fail. Depressive worries lead directly to tension in the body, and when that condition continues, it can contribute considerably to the development of cancer. We must endeavor to go about our work with a happy spirit, to do all that we can; and this will help us to keep an optimistic spirit and to enjoy nature's precious gifts with gratitude and joy. We cannot too strongly recommend the precept "Happiness Means Health."

Rule Two. We should make sure always to eat what nature offers as unadulterated, as natural, as possible. It is a proven fact that devalued, refined foods with such additives as flavoring and pesticide residues, lacking vital substances and providing incomplete protein, help to lay the groundwork for cancer.

Our diets should always emphasize alkaline foods. A lack of minerals and unsaturated fatty acids can also contribute to a degeneration of cells.

Rule Three. Do not poison your body fluids and cells with chemicals. You must understand that it is essential to avoid all therapeutic drugs that are capable of disturbing normal cell metabolism. The compulsive taking of tablets and narcotics is also responsible for upsetting the biological balance, physical as well as mental. Smokers should be aware that it is an established fact that the phenols—tar—contained in tobacco are carcinogenic.

Rule Four. One might believe that in time people will use their feet and legs only to operate the accelerator on their car. If this were so, it would present a great danger to health, robbing the body of an essential source of strength. Walking and hiking help us to breathe deeply, so that we regularly take in the oxygen the cells need to keep healthy and elastic. Cancer cells lack oxygen, and lack of oxygen is one of the main causes of cell degeneration.

Rule Five. Take great care that the cells do not experience unnecessary irritation. The liver, too, should be given constant attention and more care than other organs. The liver is the most important bulwark in the fight against cancer, and no cancerous cell degeneration is possible as long as this marvelous laboratory is working properly.

Rule Six. We know that radium and X rays present a danger to our cells, but it is also true that ever-increasing radioactivity in the environment can trigger cancer, depending on a person's predisposition and susceptibility. Limit exposure to this radiation as far as possible.

Rule Seven. The endocrine glands play an important part in our bodies and should be cared for so that they will function normally. The right balance prevents unnecessary problems. The sex glands are significant in this regard, and both excess and inhibition can be troublesome, causing irritation which is harmful to the cells. Harmony in one's married life is highly important to health in general and to cancer prevention.

Dealing with Intestinal Parasites

In the old days, when Grandmother would take a look at her grandchildren and conclude from their symptoms that they had intestinal worms, she was usually right. The children would have shadows under the eyes, pick at itchy noses, and be nervous and jumpy day and night. So what did Grandma do? She gave the children tansy or wormwood tea to drink, and later milk with crushed garlic—if stronger measures were needed, the mixture was used as an enema.

The same measures Grandmother took should be used today,

since a child who is pale, tired and moody may well have worms and should be carefully examined. Intestinal worms should never be considered harmless or their presence accepted as a necessary evil. Children with calcium deficiency are particularly prone to infestation with worms, which adds to an existing problem.

Threadworms and roundworms can cause harm by the metabolic toxins they secrete, and roundworm larvae can affect the lungs, creating a false impression of bronchitis. These worms, which can reach a length of 10 to 17 inches, can multiply in many areas of the body, dangerously obstructing the bowel or even emerging from the nose or mouth of the horrified host.

Today it has become comparatively easy to eradicate these intestinal pests with nonpoisonous plant remedies. Papaya preparations greatly facilitate the eradication of both threadworms and roundworms, actually digesting them. It is important to maintain a diet low in protein while using such preparations, as the papaya enzyme will digest the food instead of the worms.

Tapeworms are dangerous and extremely difficult to get rid of. I once helped a young man lose one by means of a diet and a special tapeworm medication, though previous treatment with chemical medicines had done him no good. My instructions for the diet and the remedy were as follows:

No meat, but plenty of vegetables and fruit, especially raw carrots, no bread, no potatoes, and nothing made of flour. For lunch, a stew of lentils, carrots, onions and garlic, cooked in one pot, perhaps seasoned with a little fresh horseradish. Twice a day a small dish of raw sauerkraut. In the morning on an empty stomach, a handful of shelled pumpkin seeds and a handful of unsweetened cranberries. Follow this an hour later with one or two cups of tapeworm tea (the recipe for which follows), without sugar. It is good to sip a glass of garlic milk as well.

Tapeworm tea. 5 grams powdered aloes, 20 grams alder buckthorn bark, 20 grams senna leaves, 25 grams valerian root, 30 grams peppermint leaves. Mix together and make an infusion, one tablespoon of the ingredients to every cup of boiling water. Brew just off the boil for ten minutes.

If no treatment whatever is able to shift the worm, an African remedy may be useful, the root of the pomegranate tree. A teaspoon of this root in powdered form should be taken in a little warm water, or two cups of tea made from boiling the root can be taken daily.

The expelled tapeworm should be burned or buried deep in the ground.

Dr. Alfred Vogel—"The Nature Doctor" in Person

For most of this century Dr. Alfred Vogel has been learning the secrets of natural healing and the curative powers of herbs, and for almost as long has shared that knowledge with patients at the clinic he ran for many years and with countless readers of his many books. Born in 1902 near Basel, Switzerland, he eagerly absorbed herbal lore from his grandparents and parents, eventually becoming familiar with the whole body of European empirical folk medicine. In later years he traveled to the remotest parts of the world, and absorbed the curative lore of tribal peoples in Africa, Asia, Australia and the Americas. His stay with the Sioux Indians in South Dakota was among the most informative and inspiring of his many tribal encounters, and gave him some literally lifesaving information as well as deepening his sense of union with nature.

At his clinic in Teufen, treatment was based on naturopathic principles, using medicinal plants gathered at the foot of the Alps, and his great interest in all methods of natural healing led him to the study and use of homeopathic treatments as well. In his worldwide lectures and the newsletter he has published for more than sixty years, Dr. Vogel has brought his experience and wisdom to many thousands, but it is his books, beginning as far back as 1925, that have carried that wisdom, and a legion of practical instructions for the full range of health problems, to countless readers in many countries. His most famous work is *Der kleine Doktor,* published in English as *The Nature Doctor,* and translated into eleven languages. Completely revised and enlarged, with exciting new information, this enduring classic of natural healing is the basis of this series of short guides to abundant health.

Dr. Vogel's decades of research and discovery have brought him professional recognition in many countries as well as the gratitude of those he has helped: he was granted an honorary doctorate in medical botany by the University of California at Los Angeles in 1952, and in 1982 was awarded the coveted Priessnitz Medal at the annual Congress of German Nature Cure Practitioners.

Though nearly ninety, Dr. Vogel still puts in a five-hour work day and attends many professional meetings and conferences, often discovering that the latest research "discovers" what he has been practicing for seven decades—and what folk medicine has known for centuries. "Only nature can heal and cure," Dr. Vogel is fond of observing, adding the corollary that "we can help and support nature and its laws that make a cure possible." This has been the basis of his lifelong work.

Bioforce: Founding and Growth. In 1963, Dr. Vogel founded Bioforce, now one of the major manufacturers of herbal extracts, homeopathic medicines, specialty health foods and biological body care products. The original production facility was located in the small farming community of Roggwil, and new ones have also been sited to allow for growth and collection of the most helpful herbs at their freshest. Experienced collectors know the best times to gather wild herbs for maximum therapeutic potency, and production employs biological methods rather than chemical or mechanical wherever possible.

Dr. Vogel is responsible for the formulations of all Bioforce products, and draws on the full range of his experience, studies and travels to assure their safety and effectiveness. Some of the most popular remedies are combinations of herbs described in booklets in this series, such as Echinaforce, Dormeasan, Crataegisan, Boldocynara, Usneasan and Symphosan, which may be obtained from herbalists or in health stores in the thirty countries Bioforce exports to.

Information on specific remedies or on Bioforce products in general may be had from the main office,

> Bioforce AG
> CH-9325 Roggwil/TG
> SWITZERLAND

or from regional headquarters:

Bioforce of America Ltd.
PO Box 507
Kinderhook, NY 12106
USA

A. Vogel of Switzerland Ltd.
1111 Gorham Street
Newmarket, ON L3Y 7V1
CANADA

Bioforce UK Ltd
South Nelson Industrial Estate
Cramlington
Northumberland NE23 9HL
UNITED KINGDOM

Bioforce Australia
PO Box 890
Eltham 3095, Victoria
AUSTRALIA

> Bioforce Singapore Pte. Ltd.
> 327 River Valley Road 03-02
> Yong An Park
> SINGAPORE 0923